ULCERATIVE COLITIS COOKBOOK

Slow Cooker

50 Easy and Tasty Low-Fiber, Dairy-Free, Nightshade-Free, Specially Designed Slow Cooker Recipes for Ulcerative Colitis, Crohn's Disease, Diverticulitis & IBD

SALLY LLOYD

CONTENT

BREAKFAST

SOUPS & BROTHS

SIDE DISH

DESSERT

Simple Plantain Mash   30

Coconut Rice Pudding   32

Pumpkin Butter   34

Blackberry Jam   36

Cranberry Orange Sauce   38

Pear Butter   40

Classic Apple Sauce   42

Coconut Yogurt   44

CHICKEN

Lemon Cilantro Chicken and Rice   46

Chicken Rice Casserole   48

Chicken Stroganoff   50

Moroccan Chicken Drumsticks   52

Pear Cranberry Squash Chicken   54

Mild Chicken Carnitas   56

Balsamic Chicken Thighs   58

Apple Acorn Squash Chicken   60

Lemon Rosemary Chicken   62

Thai Roast Chicken	64
Teriyaki Chicken	66
Fennel Orange Chicken	68
Thai Peanut Chicken	70
Bourbon Chicken	72
Chicken Tikka Masala	74
Hawaiian Pineapple Chicken	76

BEEF, LAMB AND PORK

Only for those who can tolerate

Mongolian beef	78
Beef Bourguignon	80
Classic Pot Roast	82
Italian Roasted Beef	84
Minty Lamb Shanks	86
Simple Lamb Curry	88
Apple Squash Lamb Stew	90
Lemon Rosemary Lamb	92
Honey Ginger Lime Pork	94
Maple Balsamic Pork	96
Apple Rosemary Pork Roast	98
Cuban Pork	100

BREAKFAST

OAT-STUFFED APPLES

INGREDENTS

6 green apples, top cut off and cored, leaving bottom intact

1 cup oats

1/4 cup nut butter

2 tablespoons raw honey

1 tablespoon coconut oil

1 teaspoon cinnamon

1 teaspoon nutmeg

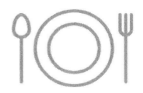

PREP TIME

5 MINUTES

COOK TIME

2 HOURS

SERVES

6

DIRECTION

1. In a medium bowl, combine all ingredients except apples.

2. Stuff apples and put into slow cooker.

3. Cook on low for 2 hours.

BREAKFAST

PUMPKIN PIE

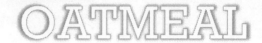

INGREDENTS

1 cup pumpkin puree

1 cup oats

2 cups water

2 cups coconut milk or almond milk

2 tablespoons maple syrup

1 teaspoon vanilla extract

1 teaspoon pumpkin pie spice

1/2 teaspoon cinnamon

1/4 teaspoon salt

  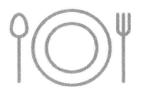

PREP TIME	COOK TIME	SERVES
10 MINUTES	8 HOURS	4

DIRECTION

1. Mix all ingredients in the slow cooker.

2. Cook on low for 8 hours.

3. Top with desired toppings and serve.

BREAKFAST

CHINESE CHICKEN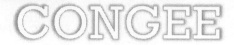

INGREDENTS

1 cup white rice, rinsed

7 cups water

1 cup chicken broth

2 bone-in chicken thighs

1-inch fresh ginger roots, peeled and sliced

Soy sauce or coconut amino for serving

PREP TIME

5 MINUTES

COOK TIME

8 HOURS

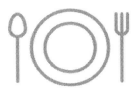

SERVES

4

DIRECTION

1. Mix all ingredients in the slow cooker.

2. Cook on low for 8 hours.

3. Remove chicken skin and shred meat. Serve with soy sauce/coconut amino if desired.

BREAKFAST

BUTTERNUT SQUASH APPLE

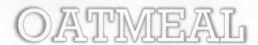

INGREDENTS

1 medium butternut squash, peeled and cubed

2 medium apples, peeled, cored and diced

1 cup coconut milk

3/4 cup almond flour (omit if can't tolerate)

1/4 cup nut butter of your choice

1 tablespoon maple syrup

1 teaspoon cinnamon

1/2 teaspoon nutmeg

Toppings of your choice

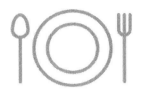

PREP TIME	COOK TIME	SERVES
10 MINUTES	8 HOURS	4

DIRECTION

1. Mix all ingredients in the slow cooker.

2. Cook on low for 8 hours.

3. Use an immersion blender or potato masher to mash into desired consistency.

4. Top with desired toppings and serve.

BREAKFAST

TURKEY BREAKFAST
CASSEROLE

INGREDENTS

1 pound lean ground turkey

1 small butternut squash, peeled, seeded and sliced

12 eggs, beaten

3 cups spinach

1 cup coconut milk

1 tablespoon coconut oil

1 teaspoon sage

1/4 teaspoon salt

PREP TIME

10 MINUTES

COOK TIME

8 HOURS

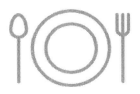

SERVES

6

DIRECTION

1. Season the meat with sage and salt. Whisk eggs with coconut milk

2. Grease the slow cooker with coconut oil. Add squash, followed by meat, egg mixture and spinach.

3. Cook on low for 8 hours.

BREAKFAST

PEANUT BUTTER
BREAKFAST BAR

INGREDENTS

3/4 cup mashed bananas

2 large eggs

1 cup oats

1 1/2 cups coconut milk or almond milk

3 tablespoons smooth peanut butter

3 tablespoons honey

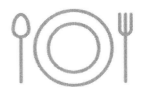

PREP TIME

10 MINUTES

COOK TIME

8 HOURS

SERVES

14

DIRECTION

1. Microwave peanut butter and honey for 30 seconds. Combine with almond milk, banana and cinnamon. Add eggs and mix well. Stir in oats and transfer the mixture to the greased slow cooker.

2. Cook on low for 8 hours.

SOUPS & BROTHS

GREEK
CHICKEN SOUP

INGREDENTS

1 pound bone-in skinless
chicken breast

3 eggs

2 stalk celery, roughly
chopped

4 cups chicken broth

2 cups water

1/4 cup lemon juice

1/2 cup uncooked white
rice, rinsed and drained

1 teaspoon salt

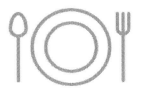

PREP TIME

10 MINUTES

COOK TIME

6 HOURS

SERVES

6

DIRECTION

1. Place chicken, celery, rice, broth, water and salt in the slow cooker

2. Cook on low for 6 hours.

3. Remove celery if can't tolerate. Shred meat and discard the bones.

4. In a medium bowl, whisk eggs with lemon juice. Spoon out a few tablespoons of hot broth and slowly stir into the lemon mixture. Then add the mixture to the soup and stir until combined.

SOUPS & BROTHS

CLASSIC CHICKEN AND RICE SOUP

INGREDENTS

2 pound bone-in skinless chicken breast

4 medium carrots, peeled and chopped

10 cups chicken broth

1 cup uncooked white rice, rinsed and drained

2 bay leaves

1/2 teaspoon dried thyme

1/2 tablespoon salt

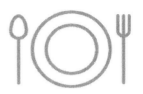

PREP TIME	COOK TIME	SERVES
10 MINUTES	6 HOURS	8

DIRECTION

1. Mix all ingredients in the slow cooker.

2. Cook on low for 6 hours.

3. Shred meat, discard the bones and bay leaves. Adjust seasoning if needed.

17

SOUPS & BROTHS

LEMONY KALE
CHICKEN SOUP

INGREDENTS

1 pound bone-in skinless chicken breast

6 cups chicken broth

1/2 cup olive oil

1 bunch kale, roughly chopped

Zest of 3 lemons

2 tablespoons lemon juice

salt to taste

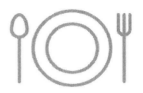

PREP TIME

10 MINUTES

COOK TIME

6 HOURS

SERVES

6

DIRECTION

1. Use a blender to blend 2 cups of broth with olive oil until it emulsifies.

2. Mix all ingredients in the slow cooker.

3. Cook on low for 6 hours.

4. Shred meat and serve.

SOUPS & BROTHS

CURRY PUMPKIN
CARROT SOUP

INGREDENTS

7 medium carrots, peeled and cut into chunks

12 ounces pumpkin, peeled, seeded and cut into chunks

4 cups chicken broth

3/4 teaspoon turmeric

1/2 teaspoon salt

1/2 teaspoon cinnamon

1/4 teaspoon ground ginger

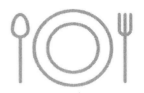

PREP TIME

COOK TIME

SERVES

10 MINUTES

8 HOURS

6

DIRECTION

1. Mix all ingredients in the slow cooker.

2. Cook on low for 8 hours.

3. Use an immersion blender to blend into desired consistency.

SOUPS & BROTHS

TURMERIC
BONE BROTH

INGREDENTS

1 whole chicken carcass

4 stalks celery, roughly chopped

2 medium carrot, peeled and roughly chopped

2 medium onions, quartered

2 sprigs thyme

2 bay leaves

2 teaspoons turmeric

1 tablespoon salt

1 tablespoon apple cider vinegar

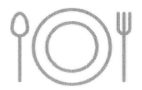

PREP TIME

10 MINUTES

COOK TIME

8 HOURS

SERVES

20

DIRECTION

1. Mix all ingredients in the slow cooker. Add enough water to cover the carcass or about an inch from the top

2. Cook on low for 8-10 hours.

3. Skim off fat from the surface. Strain the bones and vegetables using a strainer.

**The broth can be refrigerated up to a week and freeze for up to 1 month

SIDE DISH

THYME BUTTER
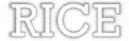

INGREDENTS

2 cups medium to long
grain white rice

8 ounces or sliced
mushrooms

4 cups chicken broth

2 tablespoons butter

1/2 teaspoon dried
thyme

1/2 teaspoon oregano

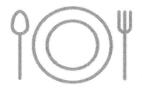

PREP TIME

15 MINUTES

COOK TIME

3 HOURS

SERVES

4

DIRECTION

1. In a pan, sauté rice with butter and herbs for 2-4 minutes. Transfer to the slow cooker.

2. Add the remaining ingredients.

3. Cover and cook on low for 2 hours. Stir and check texture. Add more broth if needed and cook for another 30-60 minutes.

SIDE DISH

BUTTERNUT SQUASH
RISOTTO

INGREDENTS

1 medium butternut squash, peeled, seeded and cut into 1/4" chunks

1 1/2 cups uncooked short grain white rice

4 cups chicken broth

1/2 teaspoon salt

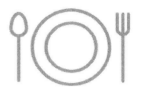

PREP TIME

15 MINUTES

COOK TIME

5 HOURS

SERVES

8

DIRECTION

1. Mix all ingredients in the slow cooker.

2. Cover and cook on low for 4 hours. Stir and check texture. Add more broth if needed and cook for another 30-60 minutes.

SIDE DISH

ROSEMARY
ACORN SQUASH

INGREDENTS

1 medium acorn squash, peeled, seeded and cut into wedges

1/2 cup vegetables broth

2 tablespoons extra virgin olive oil

3 tablespoons chopped fresh rosemary

1 tablespoon balsamic vinegar

1 teaspoon salt

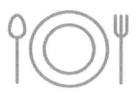

PREP TIME

5 MINUTES

COOK TIME

8 HOURS

SERVES

8

DIRECTION

1. Line the squash wedges in the slow cooker. Add broth. Drizzle with oil and vinegar. Sprinkle with salt and rosemary.

2. Cover and cook on low for 8 hours.

DESSERT

SIMPLE
PLANTAIN MASH

INGREDENTS

6 ripe plantains, peeled and cut into chunks

1 1/2 cups water

1 15-ounce can coconut milk

1/2 cup maple syrup

1/2 cup chopped almonds

1/4 cup butter

1 teaspoon cinnamon

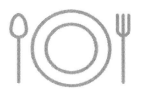

PREP TIME

5 MINUTES

COOK TIME

4 HOURS

SERVES

6

DIRECTION

1. Mix all ingredients in the slow cooker.

2. Cover and cook on low for 4 hours.

3. Serve with coconut cream if desired.

DESSERT

COCONUT

RICE PUDDING

INGREDENTS

6 cups coconut milk

1 15-ounce can coconut
cream

2 cups uncooked white
rice

3 tablespoons butter,
melted

1 teaspoon cinnamon

1/2 teaspoon vanilla
extract

1/4 teaspoon salt

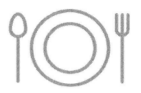

PREP TIME	COOK TIME	SERVES
5 MINUTES	4 HOURS	8

DIRECTION

1. Grease the slow cooker with 1 tablespoon butter.

2. Mix all ingredients in the slow cooker.

3. Cover and cook on low for 4 hours, stirring occasionally.

DESSERT

PUMPKIN

BUTTER

INGREDENTS

2 15-ounce cans pumpkin puree

1 cup fresh apple juice

1/2 cup maple syrup

2 teaspoons cinnamon

1/2 teaspoon ground ginger

1/2 teaspoon ground cloves

Pinch of salt

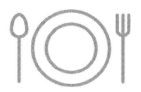

PREP TIME

5 MINUTES

COOK TIME

5 HOURS

SERVES

16

DIRECTION

1. Mix all ingredients in the slow cooker.

2. Cover and cook on low for 5 hours, stirring occasionally. Adjust sweetness if needed

DESSERT

BLACKBERRY
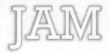

INGREDENTS

2 pounds fresh blackberries

1/2 cup maple syrup

2 limes, juice only

2 teaspoons ground nutmeg

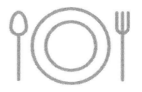

PREP TIME

5 MINUTES

COOK TIME

5 HOURS

SERVES

16

DIRECTION

1. Mix all ingredients in the slow cooker.

2. Cover and cook on low for 4 hours, stirring occasionally.

3. Cook on low, uncovered for another 1 hour until the jam thickened. Let it cool.

4. Use an immersion blender to blend into desired consistency. Adjust sweetness if needed.

DESSERT

CRANBERRY
ORANGE SAUCE

INGREDENTS

2 pounds fresh cranberries

1 1/3 cups fresh orange juice

1/2 cup maple syrup

2 tablespoons orange zest

1 teaspoon vanilla extract

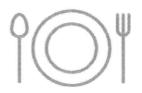

PREP TIME

5 MINUTES

COOK TIME

8 HOURS

SERVES

16

DIRECTION

1. Mix all ingredients in the slow cooker.

2. Cover and cook on low for 8 hours. Let it cool.

3. Use an immersion blender to blend into desired consistency. Adjust sweetness if needed.

DESSERT

PEAR BUTTER

INGREDENTS

2 pounds pears, peeled, cored, chopped

1 cups fresh apple juice

1/2 cup maple syrup

2 teaspoons cinnamon

1/2 teaspoon ground ginger

1/2 teaspoon ground nutmeg

1/2 teaspoon cardamom

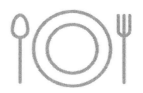

PREP TIME

5 MINUTES

COOK TIME

8 HOURS

SERVES

16

DIRECTION

1. Mix all ingredients in the slow cooker.

2. Cover and cook on low for 8 hours. Let it cool.

3. Use an immersion blender to blend into desired consistency. Adjust sweetness if needed.

DESSERT

CLASSIC
APPLESAUCE

INGREDENTS

2 pounds apples, peeled, cored, chopped

1 cups water

1/2 cup maple syrup

1 lemon, juice only

2 teaspoons cinnamon

2/3 teaspoon all spice

2/3 teaspoon clove

2/3 teaspoon ground ginger

Pinch of ground nutmeg

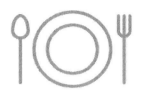

PREP TIME

10 MINUTES

COOK TIME

8 HOURS

SERVES

16

DIRECTION

1. Mix all ingredients in the slow cooker.

2. Cover and cook on low for 8 hours. Let it cool.

3. Use an immersion blender to blend into desired consistency. Adjust sweetness if needed.

DESSERT

COCONUT
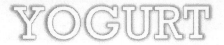

INGREDENTS

2 15-ounce cans full fat coconut milk

1 tablespoon maple syrup

2 teaspoons gelatin

2 teaspoons probiotic powder

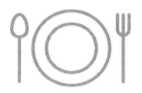

PREP TIME	COOK TIME	SERVES
5 MINUTES	15.5 HOURS	8

DIRECTION

1. Add coconut milk to slow cooker. Sprinkle gelatin on top and let it sit for 5 minutes before whisking it in.

2. Cover and cook on low for 2 1/2 hours. Then turn off the slow cooker and let it sit for 3 hours, covered.

3. Scoop out 1/4 cup coconut milk and mix with probiotic powder. Gently stir in the mixture.

4. Cover and wrap the whole slow cooker with a thick towel. Let it sit for 8 hours.

5. Transfer to a container and refrigerate for at least 6 hours before serving.

CHICKEN

LEMON CILANTRO
CHICKEN AND RICE

INGREDENTS

1 1/2 pounds chicken thighs

1 cup uncooked white rice

2 1/4 cups chicken broth

1/2 cup chopped fresh cilantro

1/4 cup fresh lemon juice

1 1/2 teaspoon salt

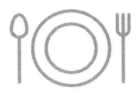

PREP TIME

10 MINUTES

COOK TIME

7 HOURS

SERVES

4

DIRECTION

1. Season chicken with salt.

2. Stir together the rest of the ingredients in the slow cooker. Place chicken on top.

3. Cook on low for 6-7 hours.

CHICKEN

CHICKEN
RICE CASSROLE

INGREDENTS

1 1/2 pounds chicken thighs

6 ounces sliced mushrooms

1 cup uncooked white rice

1 cup full fat coconut cream

1 cup chicken broth

1/4 cup water

1 1/2 teaspoon salt

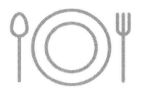

PREP TIME

10 MINUTES

COOK TIME

7 HOURS

SERVES

6

DIRECTION

1. Season chicken with salt.

2. Stir together the rest of the ingredients in the slow cooker. Place chicken on top.

3. Cook on low for 6-7 hours.

4. Shred chicken and serve.

CHICKEN

CHICKEN STROGANOFF

INGREDENTS

1 pound chicken breast

8 ounces sliced mushrooms

1 cup full fat coconut milk

1 cup chicken broth

1 tablespoon chopped fresh parsley

1 1/2 teaspoons dried thyme

1/2 teaspoon salt

  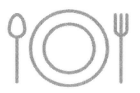

PREP TIME	COOK TIME	SERVES
10 MINUTES	8 HOURS	4

DIRECTION

1. Mix all ingredients in the slow cooker.

2. Cook on low for 6-8 hours.

3. Shred the meat and serve

CHICKEN

MOROCCAN CHICKEN
DRUMSTICK

INGREDENTS

2 pounds chicken drumstick

2 cups chicken broth

2 large carrots, peeled and diced

1 cup dried apricots, chopped

1 1/2 tablespoons grated fresh ginger

1 1/2 teaspoons sea salt

1 teaspoon cumin

1 teaspoon turmeric

1 teaspoon cinnamon

1/2 teaspoon coriander

1/2 cardamom powder

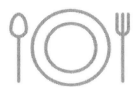

PREP TIME

10 MINUTES

COOK TIME

8 HOURS

SERVES

8

DIRECTION

1. Mix all ingredients in the slow cooker.

2. Cook on low for 6-8 hours.

CHICKEN

PEAR CRANBERRY
SQUASH CHICKEN

INGREDENTS

1 1/2 pounds chicken breast

1 medium butternut squash, peeled, seeded and diced

1 medium pear, cored and sliced

1 cup fresh cranberry

1 cup chicken broth

2 bay leaves

2 teaspoon cinnamon

1 teaspoon salt

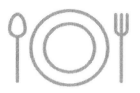

PREP TIME
10 MINUTES

COOK TIME
8 HOURS

SERVES
6

DIRECTION

1. Season the chicken with salt.

2. Layer squash in the bottom of the slow cooker, followed by chicken, pear, cranberry and bay leaves. Sprinkle cinnamon and add broth.

3. Cook on low for 6-8 hours.

CHICKEN

MILD CHICKEN
CARNITAS

INGREDENTS

1 1/2 pounds chicken breast

1 cup fresh orange juice

1/4 cup fresh lime juice

1 teaspoon ground cumin

1 teaspoon ground oregano

1/2 teaspoon salt

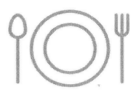

PREP TIME

10 MINUTES

COOK TIME

8 HOURS

SERVES

6

DIRECTION

1. Mix all ingredients in the slow cooker.

2. Cook on low for 6-8 hours.

3. Shred the meat and serve

CHICKEN

BALSAMIC
CICKEN THIGHS

INGREDENTS

8 boneless skinless chicken thighs

1/2 cup balsamic vinegar

2 tablespoons extra virgin olive oil

1 teaspoon dried basil

1 teaspoon dried oregano

1 teaspoon dried rosemary

1/2 teaspoon dried thyme

1/2 teaspoon salt

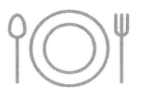

PREP TIME

10 MINUTES

COOK TIME

8 HOURS

SERVES

8

DIRECTION

1. Rub the spices and salt over the chicken thighs and place them in the slow cooker. Drizzle with oil and add vinegar.

2. Cook on low for 6-8 hours.

CHICKEN

APPLE ACORN SQUASH
CHICKEN

INGREDENTS

1 whole chicken, about 4-5 pounds

1 medium acorn squash, peeled, seeded and cut into wedges

3 medium apples, peeled, cored and chopped

1 tablespoon ground cumin

1 tablespoon curry powder (replace with 1/2 tablespoon turmeric if can't tolerate)

2 teaspoons ground coriander

1 teaspoon salt

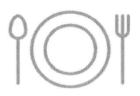

PREP TIME

10 MINUTES

COOK TIME

8 HOURS

SERVES

12

DIRECTION

1. Rub the spices and salt over the chicken.

2. Layer squash in the bottom of the slow cooker, followed by chicken. Top with apple chunks.

3. Cook on low for 6-8 hours.

4. Shred meat, discard bones and serve.

CHICKEN

LEMON ROSEMARY

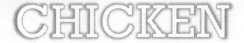

INGREDENTS

1 1/2 pounds chicken breast

1 cup chicken broth

1 lemon, sliced

5 sprigs fresh rosemary

1/4 teaspoon salt

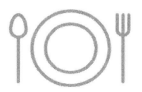

PREP TIME   COOK TIME   SERVES

10 MINUTES   8 HOURS   6

DIRECTION

1. Season chicken with salt and place the chicken in the slow cooker. Top with lemon and rosemary then pour broth over.

2. Cook on low for 6-8 hours.

3. Shred meat and serve.

CHICKEN

THAI ROAST

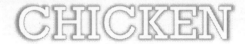

INGREDENTS

1 whole chicken, about 4-5 pounds

2 cups full fat coconut milk

3 tablespoons extra virgin olive oil

4 fresh sage leaves

2 stalks lemongrass, sliced

1 cinnamon stick

1 lemon, zest only

1 teaspoon salt

PREP TIME
10 MINUTES

COOK TIME
8 HOURS

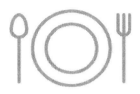

SERVES
12

DIRECTION

1. Season chicken with salt. Drizzle with olive oil. Top with lemon grass, sage leaves, cinnamon and lemon zest. Add coconut milk.

2. Cook on low for 6-8 hours.

3. Shred meat, discard bones , lemon grass, cinnamon, sage leaves and serve.

CHICKEN

TERIYAKI

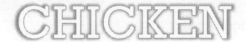

INGREDENTS

2 pounds chicken breast

1/2 cup soy sauce or coconut amino

1/2 cup honey

1/4 cup water

1/4 cup white wine vinegar

3/4 cup ground ginger

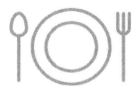

PREP TIME

10 MINUTES

COOK TIME

8 HOURS

SERVES

8

DIRECTION

1. In a small bowl, combine all seasoning ingredients.

2. Place chicken in slow cooker and pour the mixture over chicken.

3. Cook on low for 6-8 hours.

4. Shred meat and serve.

CHICKEN

FENNEL ORANGE
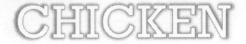

INGREDENTS

1 1/2 pounds chicken breast

3 large carrots, peeled and diced

1 fennel bulb, cored and thinly sliced

1 orange, thinly sliced

3 tablespoons extra virgin olive oil

1 tablespoons apple cider vinegar

1 teaspoon herbes de provance

3/4 teaspoon salt

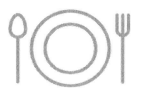

PREP TIME

10 MINUTES

COOK TIME

8 HOURS

SERVES

6

DIRECTION

1. Season chicken with salt.

2. Layer fennel in the bottom of the slow cooker. Drizzle with vinegar. Then add chicken. Drizzle with oil. Top with carrots, herbs and orange slices.

3. Cook on low for 6-8 hours.

4. Shred meat and serve.

CHICKEN

THAI PEANUT

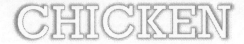

INGREDENTS

1 1/2 pounds chicken breast

1 cup full fat coconut milk

1/3 cup smooth peanut butter

2 tablespoons honey

1 tablespoon rice vinegar

1 tablespoon grated fresh ginger

1 tablespoon lime juice

1/2 teaspoon salt

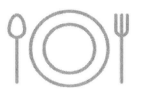

PREP TIME

10 MINUTES

COOK TIME

8 HOURS

SERVES

6

DIRECTION

1. Season chicken with salt

2. In a small bowl, combine the rest of the seasoning ingredients.

3. Place chicken in slow cooker and pour the mixture over chicken.

4. Cook on low for 6-8 hours.

5. Shred meat and serve.

CHICKEN

BOURBON
CHICKEN

INGREDENTS

3 pounds chicken thighs

1/3 cup fresh apple juice

1/4 cup soy sauce or coconut amino

1/4 cup Bourbon

1/4 cup water

3 tablespoons apple cider vinegar

3 tablespoons honey

1 teaspoon grated fresh ginger

1/2 teaspoon salt

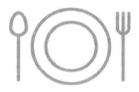

PREP TIME
10 MINUTES

COOK TIME
8 HOURS

SERVES
8

DIRECTION

1. Season chicken with salt

2. In a small bowl, combine the rest of the seasoning ingredients.

3. Place chicken in slow cooker and pour the mixture over chicken.

4. Cook on low for 6-8 hours.

5. Shred meat and serve.

CHICKEN

CHICKEN
TIKKA MASALA

INGREDENTS

1 1/2 pounds chicken breast

1 15-ounce can full fat coconut milk

1 cup chicken broth

1/2 cup chopped fresh cilantro

2 teaspoon grated fresh turmeric of 1 teaspoon dried

2 teaspoons garam masala

1 teaspoon dried coriander

1 teaspoon cumin

1/2 teaspoon salt

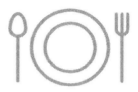

PREP TIME

10 MINUTES

COOK TIME

8 HOURS

SERVES

6

DIRECTION

1. In a small bowl, combine all seasoning ingredients.

2. Place chicken in slow cooker and pour the mixture over chicken.

3. Cook on low for 6-8 hours.

4. Shred meat and serve.

CHICKEN

HAWAIIAN PINEAPPLE

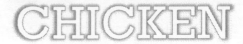

INGREDENTS

1 1/2 pounds chicken breast

2 cups fresh pineapple chunks

3 tablespoons honey

2 tablespoons soy sauce

1/4 cup maple syrup

1 tablespoon grated fresh ginger

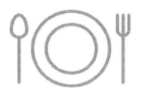

PREP TIME

10 MINUTES

COOK TIME

8 HOURS

SERVES

6

DIRECTION

1. In a small bowl, combine all seasoning ingredients.

2. Place chicken and pineapple chunks in slow cooker and pour the mixture over.

3. Cook on low for 6-8 hours.

4. Shred meat and serve.

BEEF, LAMB AND PORK

MONGOLIAN
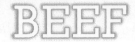

INGREDENTS

2 pounds grass-fed beef stew meat

2 large carrots, peeled and sliced

1/2 cup water

1/2 cup soy sauce or coconut amino

1/3 cup beef broth

3 tablespoons honey

2 tablespoons butter

2 teaspoons grated fresh ginger

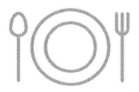

PREP TIME

15 MINUTES

COOK TIME

7 HOURS

SERVES

6

DIRECTION

1. In a pan, brown the beef in batches with butter.

2. Add browned beef and the rest of the ingredients to the slow cooker. Mix well.

3. Cover and cook on low for 6 hours. Add carrots and cook for another 1 hour.

BEEF, LAMB AND PORK

BEEF
BOUGUIGNON

INGREDENTS

2 pounds grass-fed beef stew meat, cut into bite-size

2 large carrots, peeled and sliced

1 small rutabaga, peeled and diced

2 cups bone broth

2 sprigs of fresh rosemary

2 bay leaves

2 tablespoons butter

2 tablespoons Dijon Mustard

1 teaspoon salt

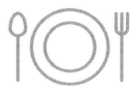

PREP TIME

15 MINUTES

COOK TIME

6 HOURS

SERVES

6

DIRECTION

1. Season the beef with salt.

2. In a pan, brown the beef in batches with butter.

3. Add browned beef and the rest of the ingredients to the slow cooker. Mix well.

4. Cover and cook on low for 8 hours

BEEF, LAMB AND PORK

CLASSIC
POT ROAST

INGREDENTS

4 pounds boneless chuck roast

1 cup beef broth

4 large carrots, peeled and sliced

2 celery stick cut into pieces (omit if can't tolerate)

2 onions, quartered (omit if can't tolerate)

1 sprig thyme

2 bay leaves

1 1/2 teaspoon salt

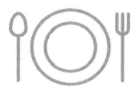

PREP TIME

15 MINUTES

COOK TIME

8 HOURS

SERVES

12

DIRECTION

1. Season the beef with salt.

2. In a pan, brown the beef on both sides.

3. Place the vegetables in the slow cooker, followed by the beef, herbs and broth.

4. Cover and cook on low for 8 hours.

5. Shred meat and serve with liquid in the slow cooker.

BEEF, LAMB AND PORK

ITALIAN
ROASTED BEEF

INGREDENTS

2 pounds beef round roast

1 small onion, sliced (omit if can't tolerate)

1/2 cup beef broth

1/2 cup red wine

1 teaspoon dried basil

1 teaspoon salt

1/2 teaspoon dried thyme

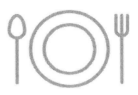

PREP TIME
15 MINUTES

COOK TIME
8 HOURS

SERVES
6

DIRECTION

1. Season the beef with salt.

2. In a pan, brown the beef on both sides.

3. Add beef broth and red wine to the slow cooker. Add the beef and sprinkle the spices on top. Top with onion slices.

4. Cover and cook on low for 8 hours.

5. Shred meat and serve with liquid in the slow cooker.

BEEF, LAMB AND PORK

MINTY

LAMB SHANKS

INGREDENTS

2 large lamb shanks

2 tablespoons butter

1 teaspoon salt

For the sauce:

1 large bunch fresh mint, leaves only

1 teaspoon apple cider vinegar

1/2 teaspoon honey

  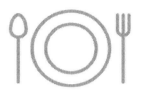

PREP TIME

10 MINUTES

COOK TIME

5 HOURS

SERVES

4

DIRECTION

1. Season the lamb with salt.

2. In a pan, brown the lamb.

3. Add lamb to slow cooker. Cover and cook on high for 5 hours. Shred the meat.

4. Use a blender or food processor to combine the sauce ingredients and serve over meat.

BEEF, LAMB AND PORK

LAMB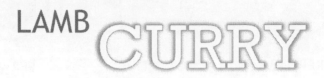

INGREDENTS

2 pounds bone-in lamb shoulder, sliced along the bones

1 15-ounce coconut milk

1/8 cup rice vinegar

2 slices fresh ginger

2 tablespoons butter

1 teaspoon salt

1 teaspoon curry powder (or replace with 1/2 teaspoon turmeric if can't tolerate)

1/2 teaspoon ground coriander

1/2 teaspoon ground cumin

1/8 teaspoon ground cloves

1/8 teaspoon cinnamon

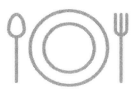

PREP TIME
10 MINUTES

COOK TIME
8 HOURS

SERVES
6

DIRECTION

1. Season the lamb with salt.

2. In a pan, brown the lamb in batches with butter.

3. Add browned lamb and the rest of the ingredients to the slow cooker. Mix well.

4. Cover and cook on low for 8 hours.

5. Shred meat and serve with liquid in the slow cooker.

BEEF, LAMB AND PORK

APPLE SQUASH
LAMB STEW

INGREDENTS

2 pounds lamb stew meat, cut into bite-size

1/2 medium butternut squash, peeled and diced

2 large apples, peeled, cored and cut into wedges

3 cups beef broth

2 tablespoons butter

2 tablespoons chopped fresh sage leaves

2 teaspoon ground ginger

1 teaspoon salt

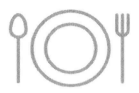

PREP TIME

10 MINUTES

COOK TIME

8 HOURS

SERVES

6

DIRECTION

1. Season the lamb with salt.

2. In a pan, brown the lamb in batches with butter.

3. Add browned lamb and the rest of the ingredients to the slow cooker. Mix well.

4. Cover and cook on low for 8 hours.

BEEF, LAMB AND PORK

LEMON
ROSEMARY LAMB

INGREDENTS

1 whole lamb leg, about 3-4 pounds

2 tablespoons olive oil

1 bunch of fresh rosemary leaves

Zest of 1 lemon

Juice of 1 lemon

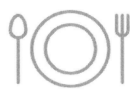

PREP TIME

10 MINUTES

COOK TIME

10 HOURS

SERVES

8

DIRECTION

1. Make incisions on the leg and stuff rosemary in it. Rub the leg with olive oil and place the leg in the slow cooker.

2. Drizzle with lemon juice and top with lemon zest.

3. Cover and cook on low for 10 hours. Shred meat and serve.

BEEF, LAMB AND PORK

HONEY GINGER LIME

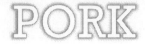

INGREDENTS

2 pounds pork tenderloin

1 lime, juice only

1/2 cup honey

1/4 cup soy sauce or coconut amino

1 tablespoon Worcestershire sauce

1/2 teaspoon ground ginger

1/2 teaspoon salt

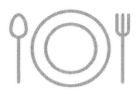

PREP TIME
10 MINUTES

COOK TIME
8 HOURS

SERVES
6

DIRECTION

1. Rub the pork with salt and place in the slow cooker.

2. In a small bowl, combine the rest of the ingredients and pour over the pork.

3. Cover and cook on low for 6-8 hours.

4. Shred meat and serve.

BEEF, LAMB AND PORK

MAPLE
BALSAMIC PORK

INGREDENTS

2 pounds pork tenderloin

1 cup water

1/2 cup balsamic vinegar

1/3 cup maple syrup

2 tablespoons soy sauce or coconut amino

1/2 teaspoon salt

  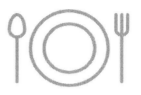

PREP TIME

10 MINUTES

COOK TIME

8 HOURS

SERVES

6

DIRECTION

1. Rub the pork with salt and place in the slow cooker.

2. In a small bowl, combine the rest of the ingredients and pour over the pork.

3. Cover and cook on low for 6-8 hours.

4. Shred meat and serve.

BEEF, LAMB AND PORK

APPLE ROSEMARY
PORK ROAST

INGREDENTS

1 whole pork shoulder roast, about 3 pounds

3 medium apples, peeled, cored and chopped

1 cup chicken broth

6 sprigs rosemary

4 sprigs basil, leaves only

1 tablespoons chopped chives

1/2 teaspoon salt

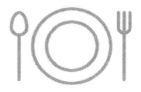

PREP TIME
10 MINUTES

COOK TIME
10 HOURS

SERVES
9

DIRECTION

1. Rub the pork shoulder with salt and place in the slow cooker.

2. Add herbs and top with apples.

3. Cover and cook on low for 8-10 hours.

4. Shred meat and serve.

BEEF, LAMB AND PORK

CUBAN PORK

INGREDENTS

1 whole pork shoulder
roast, about 3 pounds

1 small onion, sliced
(omit if can't tolerate)

1/2 cup fresh orange
juice

1/2 cup fresh lime juice

2 tablespoons extra
virgin olive oil

1 teaspoon salt

1 teaspoon cumin

1 teaspoon dried
oregano

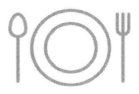

PREP TIME

10 MINUTES

COOK TIME

10 HOURS

SERVES

9

DIRECTION

1. Rub the pork shoulder with salt and place in the slow cooker. Top with onion.

2. In a small bowl, combine the rest of the ingredients. and pour over the pork.

3. Cover and cook on low for 8-10 hours.

4. Shred meat and serve.

Made in the USA
Monee, IL
04 September 2019